I0429573

*Your 30-Minute Guide to*

# Low-Willpower Eating

## The Secret to Eating Less and Weighing Less for People Who are Sick of Dieting

*Gregg Murray, Ph.D.*

To Susan and Olivia.

# TABLE OF CONTENTS

# 1. INTRODUCTION

Sick of dieting? You should be, because if you're like most overweight people, dieting leads you down a mentally difficult path of deprivation and guilt and demands a physically challenging (at best) set of rules that often actually make it harder to lose and keep off weight. *Low-Willpower Eating* provides a "secret" to eating that requires:

- Low to no willpower
- No special food

And because it makes it easier not to overeat, there are no more yo-yo weight loss and dieting. It's a "secret" that can be used for life.

Sound too good to be true? It's not. This approach is well-established in scientific circles. As a matter of fact, it is one of the top weight loss techniques of the U.S. National Institutes of Health, the American Academy of Family Physicians, and the American Dietetic Association.

*Low-Willpower Eating* is intentionally short—it is designed to be read in about 30 minutes because you are more likely to read a 30-minute guide than to finish a 200-page book. More importantly, it is a simple technique that does not require a lot of explanation or elaboration.

Read *Low-Willpower Eating*! It will free you from the physical harm and psychological pain of overeating so you can enjoy eating again.

# 2. BACKGROUND

I was the heaviest I had ever been. It was 1995, and at 5'9" and 244 pounds I was "morbidly obese." I had a beautiful wife who deserved a healthier husband and a new daughter who I wanted to see grow up. Like many "heavy" people, I had fought my weight most of my life. I didn't remember a time when eating was not an issue.

I had dieted (and almost always exercised) with some success, but I always regained the weight. Not only that, but when my dieting willpower weakened and discipline slipped, I felt like a failure and mentally beat myself up. I was sick of dieting. But at more than 240 pounds, I knew I had to do something to lose the weight. But I also knew that another round of dieting would end in the same result—losing several pounds that I regained when I began to crave forbidden food and became bored with the limited menu that I had eaten to lose weight.

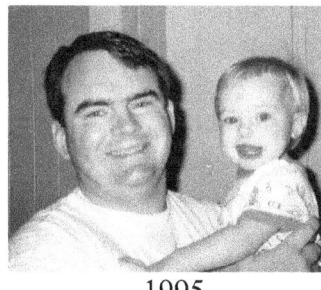

1995

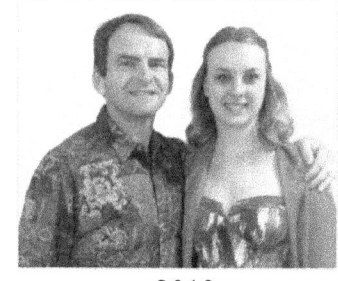

2013

I knew that to lose weight I had to burn more calories than I consumed. It was clear to me, though, that significantly restricting calories and the types of food that I ate was not going to work. It never had. And I did not have the time with my family and busy work schedule to exercise more than 30-60 minutes a few times a week. I needed a long-term, sustainable approach to eating that I could use for life. I needed something that required…

**1. Low to no willpower.**

**2. No special food.**

Just by chance I stumbled on a "secret" that met exactly those requirements: no superhuman willpower to fight constant deprivation and no unusual food(s) or limited food combinations (e.g., Mediterranean diets, low-carb or low-fat diets, high-protein diets, and even high-water content diets) to try to learn to like. I later discovered that this "secret" is well-established in scientific circles. As a matter of fact, it's on the U.S. National Institutes of Health short list of "Behaviors That Will Help You Lose Weight and Maintain It" and the American Dietetic Association's top "Ways to Shave Calories."

**The end result? I lost 53 pounds in the first year. And because this is an easily sustainable approach to eating that I have been able to maintain since 1995, I'm now over 70 pounds lighter (more than 25% of my 1995 weight) and weight is no longer an issue in my life.** I feel like I have given my wife the healthy husband she deserves, and I've treasured watching my "baby girl" grow up to be a sophomore in college this year. Thank you Low-Willpower Eating!

The rest of this guide to Low-Willpower Eating reveals the "secret" to this sustainable, long-term approach to eating less. I am a scientist who studies human behavior (in addition to my teaching duties as a college professor), so I also very briefly describe some of the behavioral science behind it. One of the keys to Low-Willpower Eating is to make it easier to avoid overeating, so this guide is intentionally short. It's a lot easier and less daunting to read a 30-minute guide than to finish a 200-page book. Besides, it is a simple technique that does not require a lot of explanation or elaboration. So the next chapter gets right to the point with the "secret" to, and specific rules of, Low-Willpower Eating.

I am confident that Low-Willpower Eating will free you from the physical harm and psychological pain of overeating the way it has freed me. Congratulations and enjoy eating!

# 3. THE "SECRET"

How many calories can you consume in 15 minutes? If you're like most people, including me, the answer is "a lot." Making a few conservative calculations using data from the U.S. Department of Agriculture's Economic Research Service indicates that in 2008 the typical American adult consumed 16 calories per minute when eating and drinking, which equates to 240 calories in 15 minutes. How significant is that? According to Harvard Medical School, to burn off 240 calories a 185-pound person requires 36 minutes of brisk walking (at 4 miles per hour), 20 minutes of running (at 12 minutes per mile), 20 minutes of cycling (at 12-14 miles per hour), 36 minutes of heavy house cleaning or gardening, or 46 minutes of grocery shopping with a cart.

*Typical Adult American, 2008:*

**2673 calories consumed per day**
**176 minutes per day eating and drinking as primary or main activity**
**16 calories consumed per minute**

So what? How is this relevant? It is relevant because 15 minutes is the amount of time it takes your brain to get the message ("satiation signals," as nutrition scientists put it) that you have eaten enough calories to sustain your body. So, many people eat for 15 or more minutes after they have already had enough to eat. And by this estimate, they could be eating 240 calories more than they need per meal.

How could this happen? It could happen if your "eating rate" (again, nutrition scientist lingo) is too fast. That is, it could happen if you "out-eat" your satiation signals. You eat so fast that your brain receives the signals that you have had enough to eat well after (15 minutes after) your body has received all the calories it needs at a meal and well after you have consumed possibly hundreds of unnecessary calories. As Ian MacDonald, Professor of Metabolic Physiology at the University of Nottingham, told BBC News for its 2008 story "Speed of Eating 'Key to Obesity'":

**"If you eat quickly you basically fill your stomach before your gastric feedback has a chance to start developing - you can overfill the thing."**

But this number is just one quick and probably overly simplistic extrapolation of some U.S. government data. Here's another piece of evidence that fast eating is associated with being overweight that uses different data, this time not just for Americans but for people in 18 economically developed countries across the globe such as Australia, Canada, France, Germany, Japan, Mexico, Poland, Turkey, and the U.S.. In a 2009 story in the *N.Y. Times* "Economix" blog entitled "Obesity and the Fastness of Food," economics reporter Catherine Rampell showed the relationship between a country's obesity rate and the average time a person in that country spends eating each day.

The graph below shows the minutes spent eating per day across the bottom (on the x-axis for you math whizzes) and the percent of the population that is obese up the left side (on the y-axis). The most obese countries (such as the U.S. at 34% and Mexico at 30%) appear in the top, left part of the graph and the least obese (such as France at 11% and Turkey at 12%) appear in the bottom, right part. The line summarizes the relationship, and its downward slope indicates that eating slower (more minutes per day spent eating) is significantly associated with less obesity.

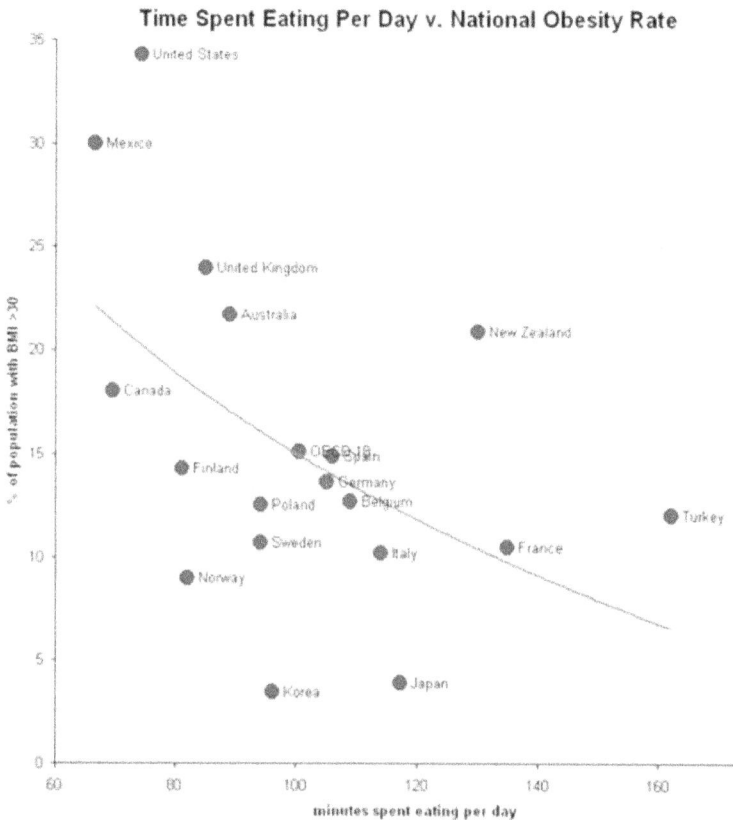

**Time Spent Eating Per Day v. National Obesity Rate**

NY Times: http://economix.blogs.nytimes.com/2009/05/05/obesity-and-the-fastness-of-food/

How about more evidence from independent nutrition scientists published in peer-reviewed scientific journals? Dr. Kathleen Melanson, PhD, RD, LD, of the University of Rhode Island and her co-authors published a study in 2008 in the *Journal of the American Dietetic Association* showing that women who ate quickly consumed 67 more calories per meal (or about 200 calories per day) than women who ate slowly. More scientific evidence…

- *International Journal of Obesity* (2003): Researchers from four Japanese universities and the Japanese National Institute of Health and Nutrition found that "Rate of eating showed a significant and positive correlation with BMI"; that is, people who ate more slowly had substantially lower levels of body fat than people who ate more quickly.

- *American Journal of Clinical Nutrition* (2009): Scientists from TI Food and Nutrition, a public-private research partnership that conducts nutrition research, found that "increasing [chewing] time significantly decreases food intake."

- *Journal of Epidemiology* (2006): Scientists from the Nagoya University Graduate School of Medicine, Japan, conclude that their "results among middle-aged men and women suggest that eating fast would lead to obesity."

- *British Medical Journal* (2008): A researcher from Harvard and colleagues showed that eating quickly is associated with being overweight for both men and women.

# 4. THE RULES

All this evidence suggests that the "secret" to eating less and weighing less without feeling deprived and without eating unusual food is to eat slowly. And Professor Ian MacDonald, our BBC News expert quoted earlier, explained that this is because when we eat too fast our brain does not receive the message in time from the "gastric feedback" process that we've had enough to eat, so we overeat. So it's that simple: **eat slowly so you can more easily tell when you've had enough to eat and you then can more easily stop eating**, not when you've eaten possibly hundreds of calories more than you actually need and want.

> **"Changing the way you go about eating can make it easier to eat less without feeling deprived. It takes 15 or more minutes for your brain to get the message that you've been fed. Eating slowly will help you feel satisfied."**

> *-- U.S. National Institutes of Health, "Get the Fullness Message"*

What are the rules? How do I "eat slowly," and how can you do it, too?

1. Put down the fork/spoon between bites.

2. Completely chew and swallow the food before taking another bite. (If you need a concrete definition of "completely chew," some suggest chewing each bite 15-20 times before swallowing.)

3. Ask yourself: "Do I feel comfortably full?" If "yes," then stop eating. If "no," then continue eating guilt free. (This is "The Deal," which you'll learn about next.)

These are exactly the rules that I use today to eat less and to avoid regaining the 70-plus excess pounds that I carried around in 1995. And because I eat until I'm full, I can enjoy food without guilt and without fighting feelings of deprivation.

**"Play 'Put the Fork Down' at meals. Put your forks down between bites and take turns sharing your day."**

*-- American Academy of Family Physicians, "Americans in Motion" Initiative*

# 5. THE DEAL

It's time to make a deal with yourself. It is the deal I made with myself in 1995 and continue to abide by to this day. This deal is the key to Low-Willpower Eating. It allows you to significantly reduce your caloric intake without requiring you to demonstrate superhuman willpower. It allows you to permanently change the way you eat. In other words, you're not on a time-limited diet to be joyously abandoned when the weight is off (and destined to be regained), you're changing how you eat permanently. Without this agreement, Low-Willpower Eating is nothing more than another diet that will help you lose a few pounds that you will gain back in the near future. Here's the deal to make with yourself:

I WILL NOT DEPRIVE MYSELF. I WILL EAT WHAT I WANT TO EAT, BUT I WILL IMMEDIATELY STOP EATING WHEN I AM FULL.

Translation: Eat the foods you regularly eat, including snacks, but stop eating when your stomach tells you that you have had enough. For example, I love Mexican food. My favorite dish is #31 at a local restaurant named "Taqueria Jalisco": a taco and two cheese enchiladas with rice and beans. Because of Low-Willpower Eating, I can regularly order and enjoy Mexican food, which is a big no-no for most diets, and neither feel guilty nor gain weight. I simply eat slowly until I am full then I stop. And I usually stop eating Mexican food, or any other meal, after about half to two-thirds of what I ate before I discovered the "secret" of Low-Willpower Eating.

But it's fair to ask, Doesn't it take willpower to stop? I'll answer that question with a question. How much willpower does it take for you to stop now when you feel full? Even when I ate fast and weighed more than 240 pounds, I stopped eating when I felt full. I didn't want any more, and I didn't want to make myself sick, so I stopped. With Low-Willpower Eating I do the same thing. I stop eating when I feel full. The difference is that before Low-Willpower Eating I didn't understand I was full until 15 or more minutes after my stomach was full, so I often ate a lot more calories than I really wanted or needed. Since I discovered the "secret," I feel my fullness much more quickly, so I avoid all those excess calories that I don't want or need.

*How do I know when I've had enough food?*

Many overweight people have a dulled ability to determine when they have had enough to eat. When this happens, it can be hard to tell if you are really hungry or if your appetite is being stimulated by other factors like boredom, emotion, advertising, a social event, the time of day, being thirsty, or a craving for a favorite food. So here are some signals of true hunger from the American Academy of Family Physicians:

• Hunger pangs, gnawing, growling, or rumbling in the stomach

• Weakness or loss of energy

• Slight headache or trouble concentrating

• Irritability or crankiness

You don't need to detect all of these signals to know it's time to eat, and you may not detect any of them. Some other signals to be aware of include:

• It's been more than five hours since your last meal

• Your last meal was very light or insubstantial

"Eat enough to satisfy your hunger and stop eating before you feel too full. There is no need to clean your plate. The goal is to feel energetic and comfortable after eating.

-- *American Academy of Family Physicians, "Americans in Motion" Initiative*

# 6. TIPS THAT MAKE LOW-WILLPOWER EATING EVEN EASIER

Many economists and other behavioral scientists like me believe that we humans often make decisions based on how much something costs relative to how much benefit we expect to get from it. For example, we won't "pay" the costs of going to a movie (e.g., expensive tickets as well as traffic, long lines, endless upcoming movie trailers, and crowded theaters) if it has poor reviews and we expect it to be a bad movie. The cost is too great relative to how much we think we will enjoy it.

Often using the same logic, nutrition scientists look at portion control. They have found that large and super-sized servings lead to overeating, which they frequently attribute to the ease (read that as "low cost") of eating those easily available additional calories. For example, I'm much more likely to eat a third enchilada at my beloved Taqueria Jalisco if I order the #31 Grande, which is a combination plate that includes a third enchilada, than if I order the #31, which has only two enchiladas. Why? Because the first two were mouth-watering, and it would take little effort to eat that third one. But if I had to get the waiter to place an order for that third enchilada then wait for it to be cooked and served to me, I'd be much less likely to eat it (and probably less likely to order it) because the effort and time to do that increase the cost of eating that third enchilada. A 2006 article in the *International Journal of Obesity* confirmed this common-sense logic. It showed that people consumed more candy from an office candy dish (68% more or more than 400 calories per week) if the dish was within their reach while sitting at their desk as opposed to six feet away.

So it helps to **increase the costs of overeating by making it harder to overeat**. How do I increase the costs of overeating, and how can you do it, too?

• Put only dinner plates, not serving plates, on the table. Increase the cost of eating more by making yourself get up from the table to get more.

• When you've had enough, remove any remaining food from the table. Take it to the sink if you're at home. Throw it out or cover it with a napkin if you're at a casual restaurant. If you're at a nicer meal, you may need to cover it with salt or sugar to "ruin" it. Remember the office-candy-dish study that showed having candy within reach led to eating more of it, a lot more of it. Removing food from the table makes it easier (less costly) to eat less.

• Don't eat out of the box or bag. Give yourself what you think is a healthy serving of whatever food you're eating then put the container back in the pantry or refrigerator. If you are still hungry after slowly eating that serving, then live up to The Deal and get more. Otherwise the cost to continue eating the food in that bag is too cheap because it's too easy to get.

• Use smaller plates. Not only does this increase the cost of eating too much because it's harder to get too much food on a smaller plate, it also increases the perceived benefit of the food because a full plate makes it look like you are getting so much more.

It also helps to **track your progress**. We behave better when we are being watched. A 1950s study of factory workers in Cicero, Illinois, showed that when factory workers thought they were being observed they were more productive, a common-sense phenomenon popularly known as the "Hawthorne" or "observer effect." As Timothy Ferriss, author of the best-selling book *The 4-Hour Body*, put it: "Seeing progress in changing numbers makes the repetitive fascinating and creates a positive feedback loop." How do I track my progress, and how can you do it, too?

• Record your weight on a sheet of paper and put it in a prominent place like on your refrigerator. Even better, make a graph using an

Excel spreadsheet—after all, a picture is worth a thousand words. This will give you positive reinforcement as you lose weight as well as serve as a reminder to check your hunger when your appetite might be stimulated by something other than true hunger. It will also increase the costs of overeating by showing you in graphic detail some of the high costs (regaining your lost weight) of overeating.

• Take and display a "before" photo. Compare this to what you see in your mirror over time to track your progress, receive positive reinforcement, and make you aware of potential costs of overeating.

For many years, my weight graph (complete with "before" picture) competed for prime space on our refrigerator with my school-aged daughter's colorful artwork.

# 7. FINAL THOUGHTS

Now you know the "secret"—and it works! Scientific evidence shows that it works. Major health organizations must think that it works because they advocate it as an important weight loss and control tool. And I am living, breathing proof that it works.

Despite all of this evidence, I am not so naïve as to think that it will work for absolutely everyone. I'm pretty sure, for instance, that if your typical meal is pizza washed down with a Pepsi and followed up with a PayDay candy bar, then you may need more than Low-Willpower Eating. Although it will help some, because you will probably know you're full well before you get to the candy bar.

Low-Willpower Eating works because it is not a diet. It is a sustainable, long-term way of eating. I am no longer sick of dieting, because I don't diet. Low-Willpower Eating does not require you to learn to eat unusual foods that you would not normally eat, and because it only requires you to do what you do now—stop eating when you are full—it does not require you to use superhuman willpower to fight food deprivation. According to the U.S. Department of Agriculture, we spend 176 minutes per day in eating activities. Low-Willpower Eating has made that time a joy for me, not torture. Thanks Low-Willpower Eating!

Get started now. Low-Willpower Eating will free you from the physical harm and psychological anguish of overeating the way it has freed me. Make The Deal then congratulate yourself and enjoy eating!

# ABOUT THE AUTHOR

Gregg Murray, Ph.D., a behavioral scientist, was haunted by food until he discovered Low-Willpower Eating. He had dieted and then regained lost weight many times in his life, but with Low-Willpower Eating he was able to lose and keep off over 70 pounds (more than 25% of his starting weight) for almost two decades now.

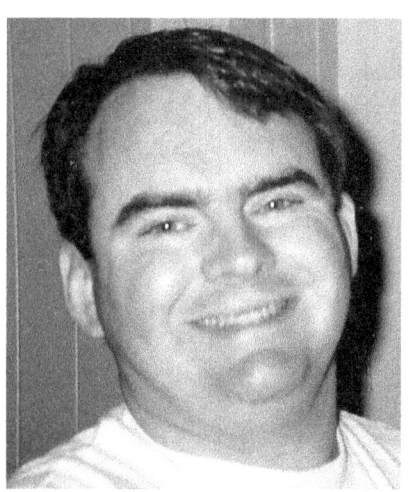
1995

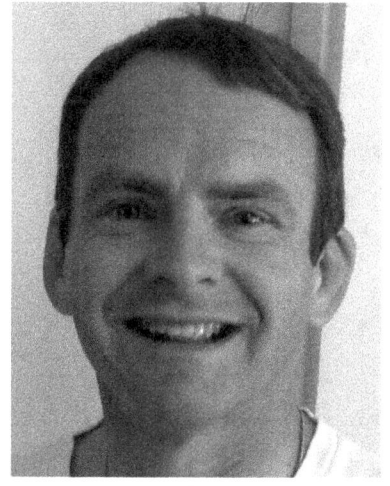
2013

How has Low-Willpower Eating worked for you? Gregg would love to hear your experiences, comments, and suggestions at LowWillpowerEating@gmail.com.